POEMS ON THE BRAIN

Sean Donnelly

Cover designed by Donna Canavan, Email: dbcbookproductions@gmail.com
About the Author photo by Jessica Snyder, Instagram: jesslaurenphoto@instagram

Sean Donnelly
Email: SeanDonnellyPoetry@gmail.com, Twitter: SeanDonnellyPoetry@poetry_sean

Printed in the United States of America

First Printing: Sep 2018
Amazon Kindle Direct Publishing

ISBN 978-1-7327714-0-6

Book Description
Do you enjoy poetry, and want to hear on a new topic? Have you ever wanted to learn about the brain, but felt bogged down with detail? If so, this is your book! Inside are 75 short and easy to memorize poems for both poetry aficionados and those studying neuroscience. The formatting has been optimized for easy flashcard use between the title and the poem.

Thank you to Kristina for being my agent and my love.

Thank you to Pablo Neruda and Ovid for inspiring me to write poetry.

Thank you to the University of New Mexico for allowing me to take my neuro courses without being enrolled in a program.

Thank you to God, my family, and everyone in my life for being amazing and making me feel welcome on this whirling speck of dust in the cosmos.

Thank you to you, dear reader, for reading my book. Please leave a review!

"To read with diligence; not to rest satisfied with a light and superficial knowledge, nor quickly to assent to things commonly spoken."

- Marcus Aurelius

INTRODUCTION

This book began in 2012 when I got into an argument with a friend. I had said that there was no interesting poetry anymore, I felt that it could be a medium to explain all of existence but it wasn't being used for that. My friend responded with a Gandhi quote, that I should, "Be the change you want to see in the world." I said, "Challenge accepted," and began to write about a topic that I was sure would never, ever get a single person to read about: Neuroscience.

Why you might want to read this book

If you enjoy poetry, this might be your jam. It's a fun and relatively arcane topic.

If you're studying the brain, this might be your jam. Each poem is 6 lines by 6 syllables, for a total of 36 syllables. You might use this as a mnemonic for memorization in your anatomy courses.

If you're not one of the first two, I'm just happy to have reached you. It's fun to be able to bring something that I consider to be exciting and beautiful to the world!

Caveat

We have fonts because Steve Jobs took a calligraphy course in college. I've taken some neuroscience courses and I have a Bachelor of Psychology. But I could be wrong... our understanding of neuroanatomy develops every day, and even something that was totally correct when I wrote it could now be wrong. You should look up each structure before you take a test on this. This is a list of those structures which I felt there was enough about to write about- some more unknown structures have been left out. This also informs on the level of detail given to individual parts, as I endeavored to say more about function than structure.

Call to Action!

If you like this book- please review it so that others will see it. If you don't- let me know and I'll improve it. In any case- thank you for reading it!

CONTENTS

AMYGDALA – CENTRAL NUCLEUS

When a kiss steals your breath
Cheeks flush with your heart's blood
And you quiver in lust
Or if you shake in rage
Or tremble in terror
Your feelings into flesh

AMYGDALA – MEDIAL NUCLEUS

Dunked in a pool, drowning
Knife's flash in dark alley
Snake's rattling in the brush
I spy sudden danger
Where Central notes delayed
The senses' door to fear

BASAL GANGLIA – STRIATUM DORSAL STRIATUM CAUDATE NUCLEUS

When life teaches lessons
When you reach for a word
I help you remember
When Love's first sight appears
When a plan is required
I prompt you to action!

BASAL GANGLIA – STRIATUM DORSAL STRIATUM PUTAMEN

A prey of Parkinson's
Dancing, playing- all taught
But I don't just move YOU
Duke of hate and disgust
I move you to ACTION
Dancing, playing...killing

BASAL GANGLIA – STRIATUM VENTRAL STRIATUM NUCLEUS ACCUMBENS

Mews and cries, lows and highs
Lover of food and drink
Addiction's creator
Dopamine dependent
Center of all wanting
Pleasure's rememberer

BASAL GANGLIA – STRIATUM
VENTRAL STRIATUM
OLFACTORY TUBERCLE

Apple pie and laundry
Printer ink and donuts
Grave dirt and baby's breath
Scents without memories
Until I do my work
Nose's link to the heart

CEREBRAL CORTEX –
CINGULATE CORTEX

In schizophrenia
I'm small and malfunction
I help you think and breathe
Desires to action
When things go right you learn
Realness known by feeling

CEREBRAL CORTEX – FRONTAL LOBE PRIMARY MOTOR CORTEX (BRODMANN AREA 4)

You Betz I'm a model
The Brain's Homunculus
My hands are very big!
Skin's motor receptors
Proxied in brain matter
Motion mapped in your mind

CEREBRAL CORTEX – GYRI INFERIOR FRONTAL GYRUS

Broca's Area's home
Names for people and things
The Linguist of the brain
Action and inaction
The fence you sit upon
Split-second course-chooser

CEREBRAL CORTEX –GYRI
SUPERIOR FRONTAL GYRUS

Face in the looking glass,
Smile, quite familiar
I tell you that it's you!
And as mirth bubbles up
That you didn't know YOU
I'm   used   in   those   laughs   too

CEREBRAL CORTEX – INSULAR CORTEX

Homeostasis Man!
Hot, cold, pulse and balance
Compassion, orgasm
Laughter, music, speaking
Your body's thermostat
Prime mover of the soul

CEREBRAL CORTEX – OCCIPITAL LOBE

Projecting in the back
A photo of your sight
What is the ventral stream?
How and where is dorsal?
Brodmann ten and seven
Visualization

CEREBRAL CORTEX – PARIETAL LOBE

Talk and mathematics
Make their home on the left
Self-orientation
Found within the right side
I tell you where you are
And describe what you find

CEREBRAL CORTEX –TEMPORAL LOBE

I remember faces
And the names of places
Episodes and items
Hippocampus encodes
While the rest of brain stores
The memory device

CEREBROSPINAL FLUID (CSF)

Saturating the brain
Providing buoyancy
No part crushing others
Cushioning from trauma
Shunting away garbage
Protective janitor

CRANIAL NERVES –OLFACTORY NERVE (1)

The first cranial nerve
I don't join the brainstem
I carry sense of smell
Though not a link to pain
Connecting nose to brain
The messenger of scent

CRANIAL NERVES – OPTIC NERVE (2)

Retina's path to brain
Blindspots at my doorway
Cross optic chiasms
Right and left meet and part
Visual cortex bound
Pathway for your vision

CRANIAL NERVES –
OCULOMOTOR NERVE (3) AND
TROCHLEAR NERVE (4)

As you focus your gaze
Or shift it not to stare
Pupils widen and close
Both eyes in unison
Eye movement messengers
Orienters of sight

CRANIAL NERVES –TRIGEMINAL NERVE (5)

Three branches from the skull
We run eyelids, sinus
Jaws, ears, mouth and forehead
No taste; but pain and heat
Letting you chew and squint
The face's puppet strings

CRANIAL NERVES -ABDUCENS NERVE (6)

Left-to-right goes your sight
My action shifting gaze
If my work is hindered
Diplopia results:
One eye sideways gazing
Eyes' right-left director

CRANIAL NERVES – FACIAL NERVE (7)

By having five branches
I innervate the face
When you smile at friends
Or wink at a stranger
I shape facial canvas
Feelings displayed in flesh

CRANIAL NERVES – VESTIBULOCOCHLEAR NERVE (8)

Link to the inner ear
Split between cochlear
Audio transducer
And the vestibular
Hairs sensing rotation
Motion and sound sensor

CRANIAL NERVES – GLOSSOPHARYNGEAL NERVE (9)

Five structures by me linked
Muscle, ear, back of tongue
Salivation and pain
Sensing bitter and sour
Coughing and swallowing
Guardian of the throat

CRANIAL NERVES - VAGUS NERVE (10)

The nervous vagabond
I have many branches
Coughing, heart-rate, hearing
Hunger and digestion
Even female pleasure
Far-ranging messenger

CRANIAL NERVES –ACCESSORY NERVE (11)

At arresting beauty
And backing out your car
Lifting up that last inch
And showing confusion
Shrugger and head-turner
Head-neck muscle-mover

CRANIAL NERVES –
HYPOGLOSSAL NERVE (12)

Talking and swallowing
Use the tongue's messenger
Shaping the words you say
Without me you would slur
Aside from the palate
Controller of the tongue

DURAL MENINGEAL SYSTEM – ARACHNOID MATTER

Spider's web to pia
Hemisphere divider
Often known with pia
As leptomeninx or
Filum terminale
CSF moving place

DURAL MENINGEAL SYSTEM – DURA MATER

DAPper from skull to brain
Sac closest to the skull
Where we end, drainage starts
Blood and CSF flow
From brain to jugular
Brain fluid reservoir

DURAL MENINGEAL SYSTEM – EPIDURAL SPACE

Natural in the spine
But not within the skull
Beyond dura mater
Canal of lymph and fat
Ending at the "great hole"
Avoid your potential

DURAL MENINGEAL SYSTEM – PIA MATER

Blood brain barrier lace
Holding the CSF
Cranial or spinal
Cushioning brain and spine
Stabilizing backbone
Shock-absorbing membrane

DURAL MENINGEAL SYSTEM – SUBDURAL SPACE

Not a thing normally
As CSF drains out
Arachnoid separates
Leaving behind a gap
Between it and pia
Artificial hollow

DURAL MENINGEAL SYSTEM – VENTRICULAR SYSTEM

Lateral: Left and right
Three horns with one body
Front, seeing, and hearing
Third: holy middleman
Fourth: boundary to spine
CSF reservoir

EPITHALAMUS –HABENULAR NUCLEUS

Rein across commisure
Lopsided left and right
Magic 8 ball of mood
Perfect for nicotine
Though many paths forward
Choosing safety from pain

EPITHALAMUS –PINEAL GLAND

Part and parcel with spine
Making melatonin
Sandman's sleep bringing draught
Formerly light sensor
Calcified brain pinecone
Timer of sleep and growth

HYPOTHALAMUS

Sleep and heat, digestion
Female orienting
Prepares milk for babies
Triggering connection
Between mother and child
And lover to lover

HYPOTHALAMUS –POSTERIOR

Remembering places
Sleep and heat controller
Hormone stops water loss
Mother's milk secretion
Triggering connection
Locator, thermostat

HYPOTHALAMUS –TUBERAL

Feeding and blood pressure
Moderating hunger
Body heat controlling
Voluntary twerking
Moderating your weight
Body regulation

METENCEPHALON – CEREBELLUM

Walking with little thought
Or reaching for something
Require no real plan
Muscles cooperate
Not fight; working as one
Motion's suave conductor

METENCEPHALON – CEREBELLUM CEREBELLAR HEMISPHERES FLOCCULONODULAR LOBE

When you maintain your gaze
All while moving your head
Independent vision
Making a sideways glance
Or fixing on a point
I free sight from posture

METENCEPHALON – CEREBELLUM CEREBELLAR VERMIS

Left-right-left, step-by-step
Delicately balanced
Tricks learned as a toddler
Control to stride ahead
Or maintain your posture
The Brain's walking center

METENCEPHALON – PARAMEDIAN PONTINE RETICULAR FORMATION

From your left to your right
Scanning the room, the page
Reading, panning, searching
With saccades, I travel
Horizontal seeing
I move your eyes sideways

METENCEPHALON – PONS PNEUMOTAXIC CENTER AND APNEUSTIC CENTER

Whether deep belly breaths
Or short-quick running gasps
I say how fast you breathe
From long sighs to hot puffs
Phrenic's inhibitor
Modulators of breath

METENCEPHALON – PONS
CRANIAL NERVE NUCLEUS

Nerves 5,6,7,8!
White matter within gray
Brain nerve passage between
Your midbrain, medulla
And your cerebellum
Your bridge of Varoli

MIDBRAIN – PRETECTUM

Dilating your pupil
Filtering light inside
Tracking sudden motion
On quick change, I focus
Tracker and gatekeeper
Movement and light tracker

MIDBRAIN –TECTUM

Directing where you look
And where you reach towards
I combine your senses
Their inputs into one
Inner map of the world
Directing your action

MOTOR SYSTEMS –ALPHA MOTOR SYSTEM

Alpha Motor Neurons
Innervating by height
Many for more detail
Bonding muscle and brain
Without us no motion
Chosen or by reflex

MOTOR SYSTEMS – EXTRAPYRAMIDAL SYSTEM

My methods indirect
No innervation here
To lower spinal cord
I suggest my orders
Conductor of movement
Syncing many motions

MOTOR SYSTEMS –GAMMA MOTOR SYSTEM

I keep your muscles tight
Able to move quickly
Static for more control
Dynamic for quick change
Awareness of their place
Preparer of action

MOTOR SYSTEMS −PYRAMIDAL TRACTS

Counter puppeteering
Right side controlling left
Nerves encased in sheathes
Cortex to the body
Movement control
There are some strings on you

MYELENCEPHALON –MEDULLA OBLONGATA

Wheezing and swallowing
Knowing to gasp for air
And the pumping of blood
Reflex, blood and breathing
Bottom of the brainstem
Oxygen manager

NEURAL PATHWAYS -ARCUATE FASCICULUS

Wernicke's and Broca's
Expression of one's mind
Comprehension of words
Together by me linked
Musical tone as well
Pathway from speech to thought

NEURAL PATHWAYS -CEREBRAL PEDUNCLE

Brain path from high to low
Midbrain minus tectum
Not gray, nor white, but black
Handling mood and movement
Of body and the eyes
Dark pathway to motion

NEURAL PATHWAYS -CORPUS CALLOSUM

Main road from left to right
Chain free thought to logic
Messages between halves
Coordinate action
Emotion with process
Fantasy to logic

NEURAL PATHWAYS – CORTICOSPINAL AND CORTICO BULBAR TRACTS

Through me mirrored movement
Sent from brain to body
Traversing white matter
–Spinal and –Bulbar tracts
Connect mind to corpus
Form and face meshed to brain

NEUROENDOCRINE SYSTEMS – HYPOTHALAMIC-PITUITARY-ADRENAL AXIS

Stress response feedback loop
Waking with cortisol
Calming immune response
Balancing life's stressors
With learned or innate acts
Preserving from danger

NEUROENDOCRINE SYSTEMS – HYPOTHALAMIC-PITUITARY- GONADAL AXIS

Sex hormone feedback loop
Started at puberty
And ending at old age:
For women, menopause
For men, reduced function
Sexual on/off switch

NEUROENDOCRINE SYSTEMS – HYPOTHALAMIC–PITUITARY–THYROID AXIS

Gluttony feedback loop
Less thyroid, more famished
Pituitary halts
Your stomach growls at you
Sensing that you need food
Hunger-sating system

PITUITARY GLAND

Lord of the nine hormones
Food metabolism
Body temperature
Teenage growth spurts and sex
Pregnancy, Childbirth
Chemical thermostat

PREFRONTAL CORTEX – DORSOLATERAL PREFRONTAL CORTEX (BRODMANN 9 & 46)

Selfless sense of fair play
Commitment to your love
And the critic of dreams
I give a sense of right
In actions or events
Your ruler and ruler

PREFRONTAL CORTEX – ORBITOFRONTAL CORTEX (BRODMANN 10,11, & 47)

Urge to safely achieve
Grasping gain through the rules
Fearful of consequence
Guarding through rituals
The foe of addiction
Fear/pleasure balancer

PREFRONTAL CORTEX – VENTROMEDIAL PREFRONTAL CORTEX (BRODMANN 12, 44, 45, & 47)

Wisdom of adulthood
Over folly of youth
I teach impulse control
While you may know what's right
I guide you to DO it
Righteous shoulder-angel

RHINENCEPHALON -ANTERIOR COMMISURE

Second-string messenger
(Save in marsupials)
Between Amygdalas
And R/L hemispheres
Of sharp pain and hearing
Memory, sex and smell

RHINENCEPHALON -OLFACTORY BULB

Smell categorizer
I keep an odor map
Sorting one from many
I amplify the faint
Warn of spoilage and rot
Telling you each scent's name

SUBCORTICAL – BASAL GANGLIA GLOBUS PALLIDUS AND SUBTHALAMIC NUCLEUS

The sleekness of dancing
And swift music of speech
I'm motion's lubricant
Removing jerkiness
Smoothing each of your steps
Greasing every gesture

SUBCORTICAL – CLAUSTRUM

A brown disc, silver wrapped
Apple scent, syrup taste
To know its apple pie
Is knowledge I provide
Sensing integrator
The seat of consciousness

SUBCORTICAL – HIPPOCAMPUS

I take notes as you go
Of what happened today
But who recalls your wife?
Or how to play the flute?
It is a mystery
Author of life events

THALAMUS – ANTERIOR NUCLEI

Doorway to memory
Being in the moment
Actively turning heads
Directing attention
Events written in stone
Observation concrete

THALAMUS – MEDIAL NUCLEAR GROUP

Short-term memory base
Attentive task switcher
Stressing but quick-thinking
Fear and senses binder
System integrator
Active first responder

THALAMUS – METATHALAMUS

Visual field combined
Backwards fields, left and right
Left getting less than right
Vision subdivided
Right getting past the nose
Vision across the eyes

THALAMUS – VENTRAL NUCLEAR GROUP

Mapping and controlling
Motion and location
Feeling skin sensations
Itching, pain, tingling
Locator of oneself
And what one feels while there

VASCULAR SYSTEMS – BLOOD-BRAIN BARRIER

Semi-permeable
Blocking for CSF
Molecules and cells stopped
While Transport proteins let
A select few across
Bodyguard of the brain

VASCULAR SYSTEMS –CIRCLE OF WILLIS

Circle from carotid
Back to cerebellum
Though quite often malformed
With blood sometimes stolen
Backup blood supplier
Brain's arterial source

WHITE MATTER – ARCUATE FASCICULUS

Broca to Wernicke
Speech to understanding
Knowing what you're saying
Whether hearing a note
Or speech without stutter
Translating sound to thought

WHITE MATTER –CORONA RADIATA

Projection fiber sheet
Each site matched to body
Information highway
Back and forth from cortex
Nerves wrapped in myelin
Brain–body address book

WHITE MATTER – UNCINATE FASCICULUS

Growing past age thirty
Right side for social trust
And processing your past
Left side for intellect
And fact-based memory
Eventual morals

BONUS CONTENT - PREVIEW

Monoamine Neurotransmitters

MONOAMINE NEUROTRANSMITTERS – DOPAMINE

Chemical messenger
Substantia nigra born
Action threshold setter
Too much brings psychosis
Too little causes pain
Impulsiveness benchmark

MONOAMINE NEUROTRANSMITTERS – SEROTONIN

5-HT receives me
Uptake stops my action
But if I'm left alone
Then I will get you high
Pain, fullness, and drug highs
Controller of good times

MONOAMINE NEUROTRANSMITTERS – HISTAMINE

Asleep versus awake
Set by rate of fire
Faster to be alert
Slower towards dreamland
Stimulating mucous
Sleepy and sneezing dwarves

MONOAMINE NEUROTRANSMITTERS – EPINEPHRINE (ADRENALINE)

Adrenal gland produced
Fear induced secretion
No down-regulation
Memory enhancer
Berserker strength hormone
Fight or flight, get pumped up!

MONOAMINE NEUROTRANSMITTERS – NOREPINEPHRINE

Sympathetic to stress
Maintenance to action
No sleep or digestion
Freeing up energy
To ensure survival
Vigilant defender

ABOUT THE AUTHOR

Sean Donnelly is a managerial accountant. He received his bachelors in Psychology, took 6 credits of neuroscience at the masters level, achieved his Masters in Accounting, and is working on his Doctor of Business Administration. In other words, he's not a professional neuroscientist, but an amateur poet writing about the brain. He enjoys computer games (League of Legends, Overwatch, Heroes of the Storm, etc.) and loves to read textbooks. If you have enjoyed this book, he'd love to hear about it. He'd love a positive review on Amazon.com too. If he's wrong in any particular poem, or you hate this book, he'd love to hear that too. Pending verification, he'll fix any errors/updates in the next edition. Thank you!

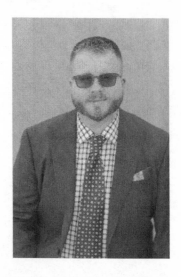

Email: SeanDonnellyPoetry@gmail.com
Twitter: SeanDonnellyPoetry@poetry_sean

REFERENCES

Kandel, E. R., Schwartz, J., & Jessell, T. (2000). *Principles of Neural Science (4th ed.).* NY, NY: McGraw-Hill Medical.

Langley, L. L., M.A,PH.D., & Cheraskin, E., M.D.,D.M.D. (1954). *The Physiology of Man.* New York, NY: McGraw-Hill Book Company.

Neruda, P., & Tapscott, S. (2000). *100 Love Sonnets = Cien Sonetos de Amor.* Austin, TX: University of Texas Press.

Netter, F. (2004). *Atlas of Human Anatomy (3rd ed.).* Teterboro, NJ: Icon Learning Systems.

Made in the USA
Lexington, KY
28 January 2019